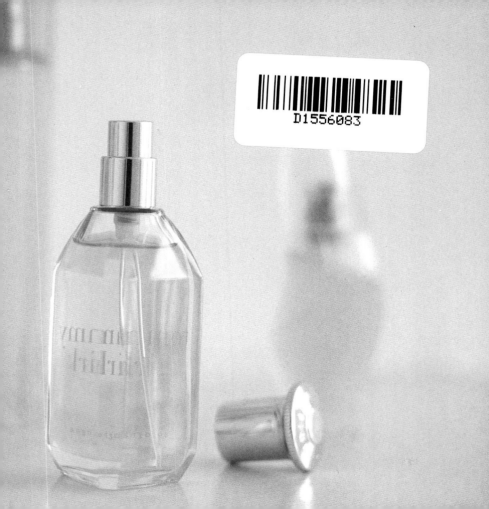

A PASSION FOR *perfume*

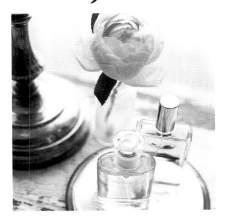

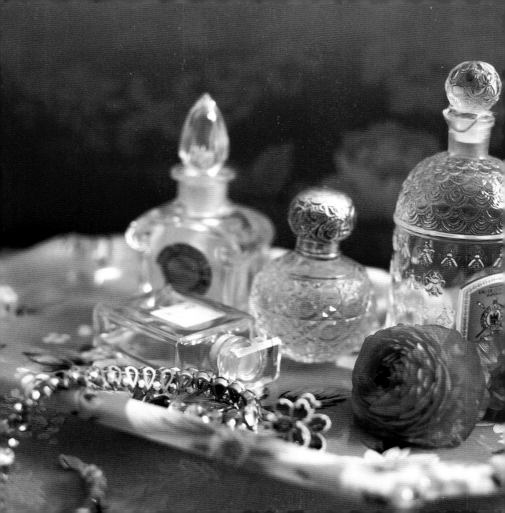

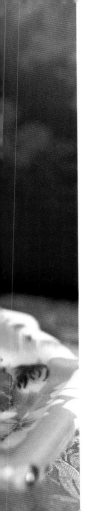

A PASSION FOR
perfume

Jo Glanville-Blackburn
photography by Claire Richardson

RYLAND
PETERS
& SMALL
LONDON NEW YORK

Designer Pamela Daniels
Editor Miriam Hyslop
Location Researcher Tracy Ogino
Production Gemma Moules
Art Director Gabriella Le Grazie
Publishing Director Alison Starling
Stylist Twig Hutchinson

First published in Great Britain
in 2005 by Ryland Peters & Small
20–21 Jockey's Fields
London WC1R 4BW
www.rylandpeters.com

10 9 8 7 6 5 4 3 2 1

Text © Jo Glanville-Blackburn 2005
Design and photographs
© Ryland Peters & Small 2005

The author's moral rights have
been asserted. All rights reserved.
No part of this publication may be
reproduced, stored in a retrieval
system, or transmitted in any form
or by any means, electronic,
mechanical, photocopying or
otherwise, without the prior
permission of the publisher.

ISBN 1 84172 977 9

A CIP record for this book is
available from the British Library.
Printed in China

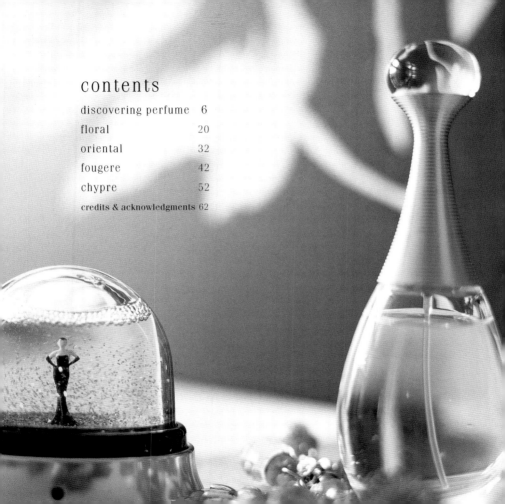

contents

discovering perfume

Perfume is the one thing that we leave as an imprint of ourselves, always living in the memory of others.

Scent is essential to our life and to our wellbeing. Whether it's the aroma of a favourite flower, the comfort of wood-smoke next to Father's old pipe, or the heavenly scented kiss curl at the nape of your baby's neck, scent matters.

Our sense of smell is the sense most linked to memory and emotion and is the sense that we instinctively trust the most. Smell triggers emotions both good and bad. That's why perfume matters, for if you have a positive association with your chosen scent you will have your ultimate therapy in a bottle.

Beyond photographs, the one thing that keeps the memory of my late mother alive is her scent. From the moment I smell her perfume – the very bottles that she had adored that are, quite simply, 'Mummy' – I have comfort, her arms around me. In her perfume, I can still conjure up the image and memory of every hug and kiss we ever shared.

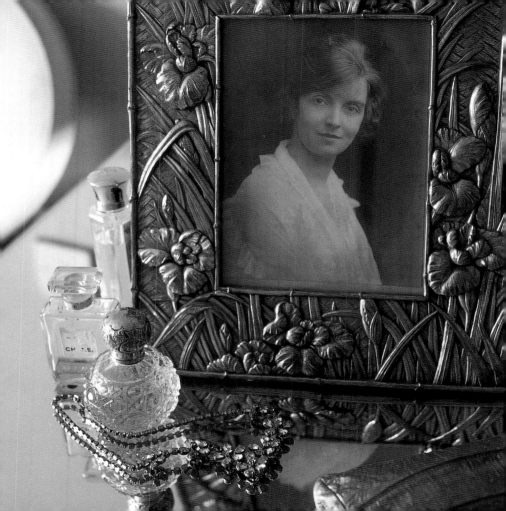

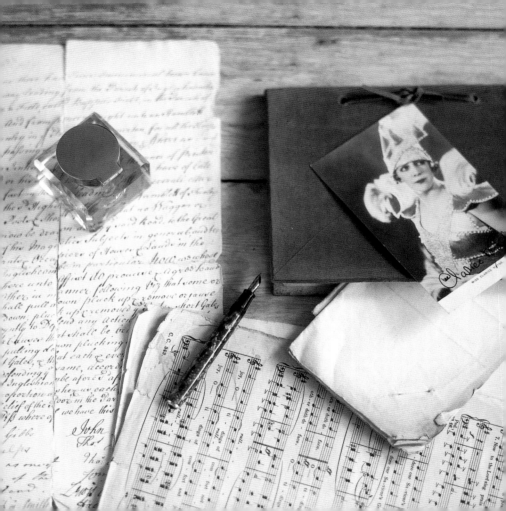

scent & memory

For many, a single waft of rose puts us back among the summer rosebeds of our childhood. For others, the smell of freshly mown grass rekindles youthful days living in the countryside, and cinnamon conjures Christmas.

Scent captures our memories and holds them dear. Unlike the other senses, smell channels fragrance directly to the brain's limbic system, the part of the brain that is home to our memory, emotion and imagination. It's potent stuff. That's why scent triggers memories and why perfume is like an opiate to the soul, holding great power over us.

According to aromachologists and perfumers, however, the way that scent and memory are linked defies logic. While a single aroma of rose, lavender or apple might trigger a number of associations for us all, some scents are not as pure. Johnson's baby oil, for example, contains over 120 different ingredients, yet our sense of smell recognizes the aroma and places in our heart alongside baby's bathtime or our own childhood.

Scent has the ability to conjure up sweet memories and bring back a solitary, single moment in your past with startling clarity and emotion.

scent & personality

When you wear perfume the scent is with you for the entire day, and whoever you meet might build their own image of you based on the way you smell. By choosing a particular scent, you ensure that you are surrounded by the things that make you unique – and the things that you love. Your choice of perfume can reveal the 'real you'.

Perfume heralds a woman's arrival and prolongs her departure.

COCO CHANEL

Perfume reflects our personality. Scent psychologists can predict the type of scent an extrovert might choose over an introvert, and blondes tend to opt for different scents to brunettes and redheads. Subtle differences in the acidity of the skin is one reason why scents smell differently on us all. But other factors such as diet, health and hormones influence our body chemistry, too.

Ultimately choosing a perfume because of how it makes you feel – whether for comfort (vanilla), energy (rosemary), or to make you feel pretty (rose) – is a great way to select the right one for you. 70 per cent of our values, likes and dislikes come from our experiences in childhood. If, for instance, you

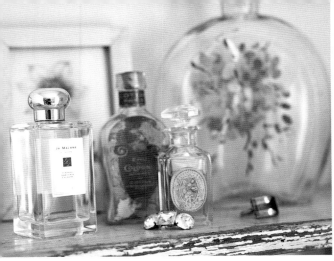

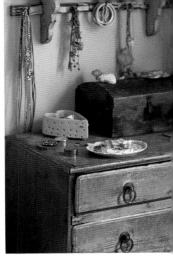

have wonderful memories of your mother wearing rose and kissing you goodnight, chances are, whenever you smell rose, you will feel uplifted and happy. The smell of leather might remind you of an old car, music lessons (my old tattered, much-loved music bag smelt like heaven) or Daddy's desk. Mood-altering fragrances are simply scents that instil uplifting feelings of joy, happiness, serenity, allure – all things positive. Aromatherapy is the ultimate mood-enhancing aromatic therapy, so perfumery is the aromatherapist's dream job.

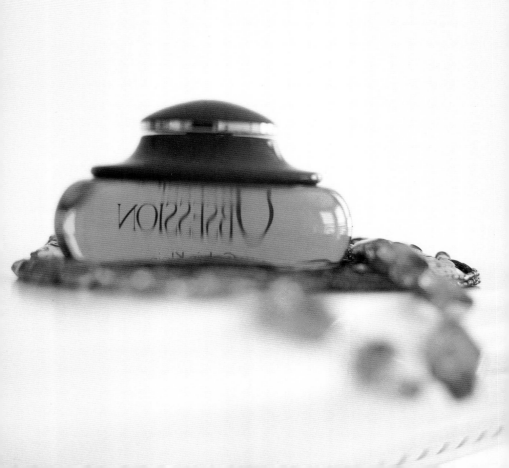

scent & seduction

What remains of a woman when she is in the dark? When she has undressed, when we can no longer see her make-up, her wonderful hair, her beautiful eyes, when she takes off her jewellery, what is left? Only her charming voice and . . . her perfume.

JEAN-PAUL GUERLAIN

Fragrance is a sensory language. It can be a potent seducer that works on a very fundamental level.

∞ 1940s Hollywood movie star Joan Crawford was wearing Youth Dew (a rich opulent fruity oriental) when she met her husband, Alfred Steele. 'I can't stop dancing with you,' he said. 'You smell exquisite.'

∞ Cleopatra first met Mark Antony on her royal barge, upon which the purple sails were drenched in her perfume.

∞ Marquise de Pompadour fixed tiny scented stars about her person for Louis XV to delight in finding.

scent composition

Making a perfume is like the theatre: you might have the actor but without the props, music and lights, it won't work. So you work on the production until it becomes mesmerizing, but never losing sight of the real performer.

JO MALONE

There are four traditional fragrance families: floral, oriental, chypre (pronounced 'shee-pray') and fougere. These signify the key notes in each of the four main fragrance families. Within each family there are smaller families or subdivisions (for example, a flori-oriental or fruity chypre) where other notes, such as lively citrus or popular mouthwatering fruity notes, add a twist and take each fragrance to another level. These fragrance families are ever-expanding and evolving, with new ingredients (though now often synthetic) being created every day. They are the best basis for choosing and understanding why you might prefer one fragrance to another.

Generally, fragrances are composed using the principle of three categories of 'notes' of varying intensities to balance them in a lasting aroma. The more top notes there are (eau de Cologne, then eau de toilette), the quicker the fragrance will disappear. The more base notes (perfume), the longer the scent will last.

top notes

Top notes are the first to strike
but are ephemeral (think citrus,
herbal fresh and fougere).

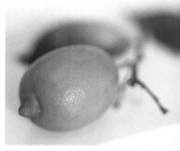

middle notes

Typically 50–80 per cent of the
blend, middle notes linger longer
and make the heart of the scent
(think pretty lasting floral).

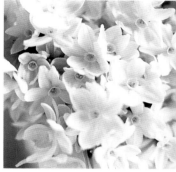

base notes

Base notes, or 'fixatives',
provide lasting woody or animal
notes that stabilize the entire
blend. This part of the fragrance
lasts the longest on your skin
(think evocative rich oriental
and chypre).

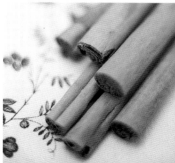

how to choose a scent

Never go with a friend. Fragrance is so personal, and such a reflection of our own being and our own personality, they may well force their own tastes on you. It could be a relationship that lasts a lifetime — the perfume, that is!

ROJA DOVE

Choosing a new scent is very personal, and the decision should never be rushed.

∞ Don't wear perfume when choosing a new one.

∞ Avoid shopping for scent after eating a spicy meal, as the chemistry of your skin may alter the aroma.

∞ Never choose a fragrance because it smells good on someone else. It may well not smell the same on you.

∞ Don't judge a scent in the bottle. You'll only smell the transient top notes and the alcohol that it is diluted in, not how it will smell on your skin. Think of your skin as the final essential ingredient in a fragrance.

∞ Spray and walk away for an hour. You may love the top notes, but it is the base that determines the final aroma on your skin, and this takes about an hour to develop. This is the time to make your decision.

∞ Avoid smelling too many scents at once – just try three or four at any one time. You can try wafting coffee beans under your nose to cleanse and refresh your smelling powers.

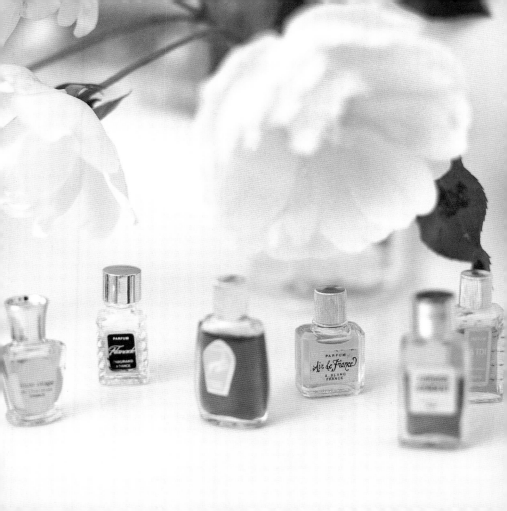

Always apply perfume in the dip of the collarbone (not behind your ear), because the first thing someone does when they're getting closer and more intimate is to whisper in your ear. This way their nose is directly over the 'hot spot', and if your chosen scent contains the necessary aphrodisiac, the magic will be there.

ROJA DOVE

how to wear it

*Apply perfume
wherever you
want to
be kissed.*

COCO CHANEL

✿ Layer fragrance to make it last longer. Always use bath oils and body moisturizers that match your perfume. Apply scent before applying body moisturizer – by applying the cream last, you seal the fragrance next to your skin, where it works magic with your body chemistry. This makes it last longer, too.

✿ When you apply perfume, always use the stopper (bottles are better than sprays – you use less). Once used, wipe clean using a small silk square. The oils from your body and dead skin cells will otherwise go into the liquid and ruin its integrity. Silk has a magical property of being able to hold perfume – then you can drop it into your lingerie drawer to delicately scent your clothes, or even in your luggage while you are travelling, so everything will smell nice when you open it.

✿ The inner crook of the elbows and the inside of the wrists are the perfect place to apply perfume if you're a 'draping' kind of female. Alternatively, if you are sitting for dinner or cocktails, the ankle or behind the knee is perfect as the perfume rises in the heat. In Eastern tradition, the navel is a popular place to apply perfume, so that later, if he travels lower…

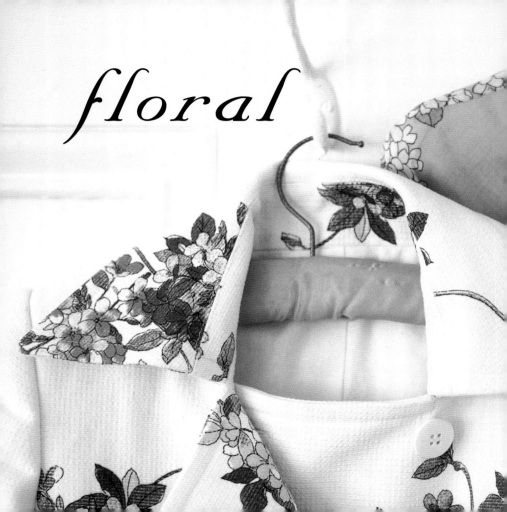

floral

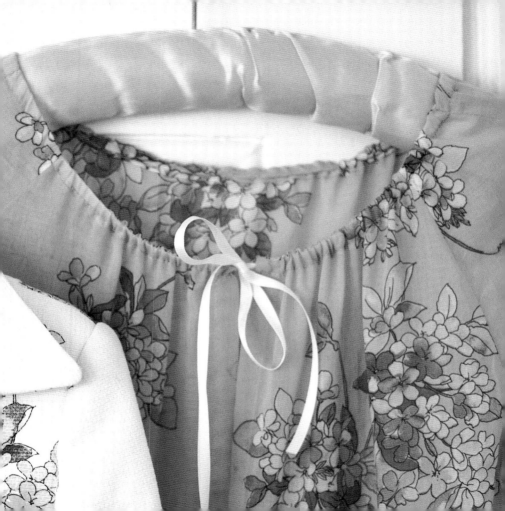

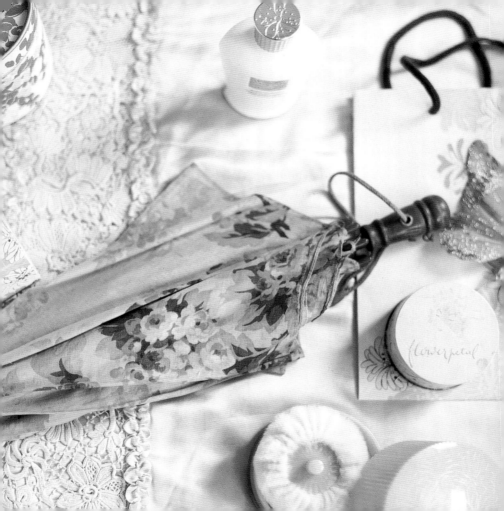

petal soft

Walk through a garden after the rain and you can smell flowers in their virgin state: pure, clean and vibrant. It's beautiful. Some flowers are brash and let you know they're there in the late evening light. Others draw you close, begging to be caressed.

From the very moment you pick a flower, its chemistry changes. In perfumery, roses need to be picked at sunrise and processed within 24 hours to truly capture their scent. Each bush takes four years to mature and can bear over 400 blossoms. Every rose-picker collects between 2,000 and 3,000 petals in an hour – the equivalent of four tiny drops of precious rose absolute (pure essence) – which makes it one of the most expensive oils to produce.

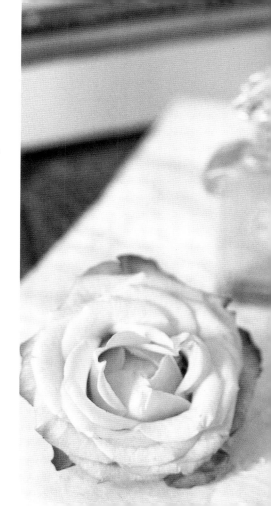

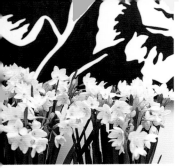

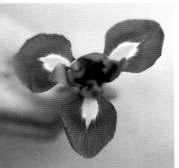

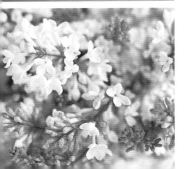

Women need floral scents. Flowers translate affection, delicacy, happiness and beauty. Florals are the emblematic sign of femininity and create scents that talk to the heart. Warm exotic florals such as tuberose, jasmine and ylang-ylang are more sensual, while simple flowers, such as rose, are fresh.

Florals are the largest of the four fragrance families, accounting for nearly two-thirds of all fragrances ever made. As a general rule, those who like floral perfume will have sunny, carefree dispositions. Women who like florals with freshness tend to look to the future, whilst those who prefer powdery florals (such as orris) are more romantic and nostalgic. The lover of white florals adores the idea of being sensual, but would never be so brazen as to wear an oriental scent.

Perfumers believe that any love potion needs a medley of exotic white flowers. This may be because they contain a magical molecule called indole (found naturally in the genitals and armpits), which occurs naturally in musk and arouses the base and animal instincts in us all.

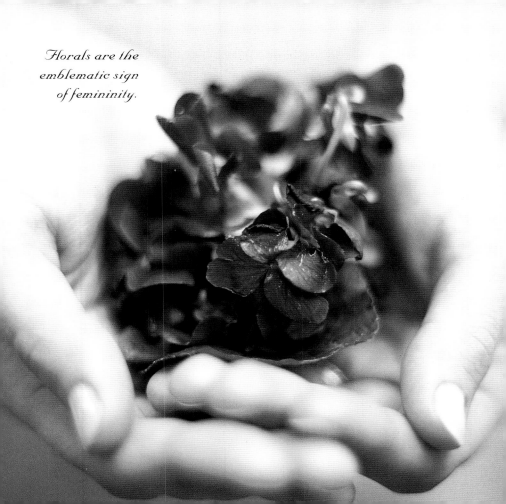

*Florals are the
emblematic sign
of femininity.*

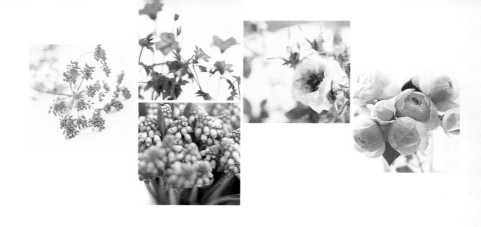

ingredients & notes

Exotic floral notes are heavily, overtly scented and, more often than not, tend to be white fragrant flowers.

Heavily scented fragrant flowers are used in perfumery to suggest excitement and sensuality. Excluding the rose, most intensely fragrant flowers are white. Think gardenia, honeysuckle, lily-of-the-valley, ylang-ylang, and of course the queen of flowers, jasmine. Found in a garden, these flowers have no colour to attract bees and other insects to them for pollination and so rely entirely on their intoxicating scent for chemistry. Which is one good reason why you'll often find them in some of the sexiest fragrances ever made.

LILY OF THE VALLEY This
exerts its charm under the
early evening sun. Legend
tells us that the small white
bell-like flowers were formed
from the tears of the Virgin
Mary, thus making the floral
infusions so valuable in the
Middle Ages that they were
kept in gold and silver vessels.
Through this the plant later
acquired another name,
'ladder to Heaven', hinting at
the sleep of divine dreams.

ORANGE BLOSSOM In
ancient history, orange
blossom symbolizes innocence
and purity, and newlyweds
would fill their bouquets with
the flower.

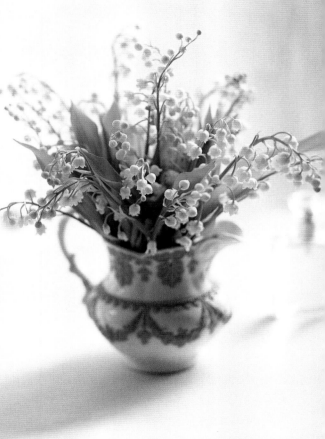

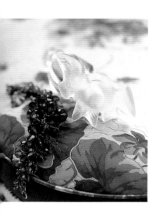

ORRIS An expensive and important note in perfumery. Its soft powdery aroma – similar to violet – mingles perfectly with the skin and adds a touch of deep woody softness and warmth. Orris root is the name given to the root of the iris plant, and it has been prized in perfumery since the ancient Greeks because of its violet scent. In the Middle Ages, orris formed the base of many perfumed preparations for the hair, body and laundry, and it was made into rosary beads.

JASMINE The intense narcotic perfume of jasmine is the most popular floral absolute (pure essence) still used today in perfumery. The tropical flowers radiate peak potency on warm sultry evenings, giving it the Indian name of 'Moonlight of the Groves'. In the East, whole streets are given over to jasmine flower sellers, seen threading the blooms for local women to perfume their hair or to offer to the gods. The flower essence has a deep, warm, creamy encompassing perfume with fruity green undertones, which becomes more seductive on contact with the skin. It requires eight million jasmine blossoms to make just 1kg of pure essence, making it one of the most expensive flowers in perfumery, alongside rose, neroli and tuberose.

Flowers are magical. They're the heart of a fragrance, and a fragrance without a heart has no soul.

LYN HARRIS, PERFUMER

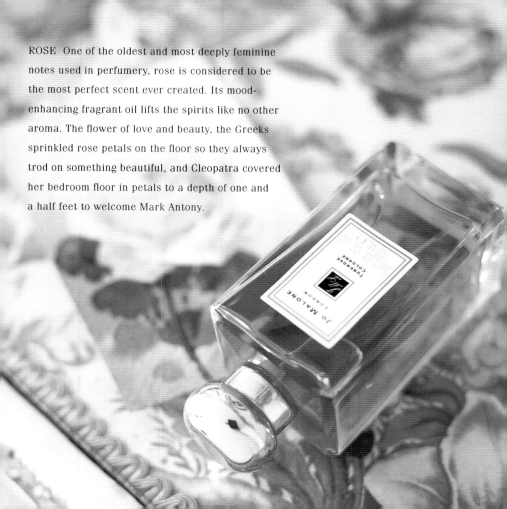

ROSE One of the oldest and most deeply feminine notes used in perfumery, rose is considered to be the most perfect scent ever created. Its mood-enhancing fragrant oil lifts the spirits like no other aroma. The flower of love and beauty, the Greeks sprinkled rose petals on the floor so they always trod on something beautiful, and Cleopatra covered her bedroom floor in petals to a depth of one and a half feet to welcome Mark Antony.

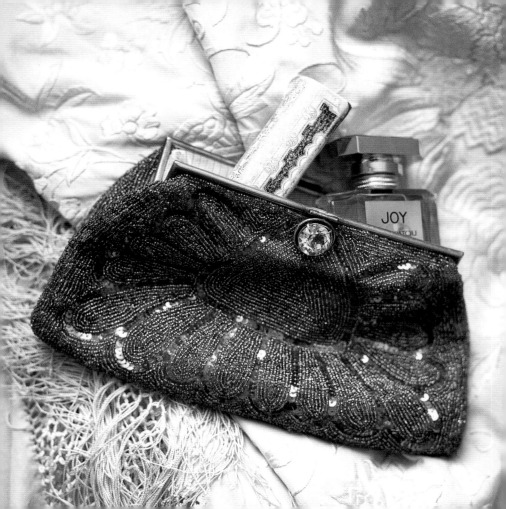

classic floral

JOY BY JEAN PATOU

First available in the late 1920s, around the time of the Wall Street crash, Joy was the perfect antidote to a depression. A hefty blend of Damascene rose, rose de Mai and jasmine from Grasse, it established itself as 'the costliest perfume in the world', yet it still ranks in the top five best-selling perfumes of all time. It takes over 10,000 jasmine blooms and 28 dozen roses to make a single fluid ounce of Joy.

Two legends united: Marilyn Monroe once said that all she wore in bed was No 5.

CHANEL NO 5

This bouquet of abstract flowers was the first fizzy aldehydic (sparkling) floral in perfume history. Today, No 5 is still the world's number one best-selling woman's fragrance. Its code name and winning number, the number 5, corresponds to the fifth prototype chosen by Coco Chanel. It was also her lucky number: all her collections were shown on the fifth day of the month, and the fifth month of the year.

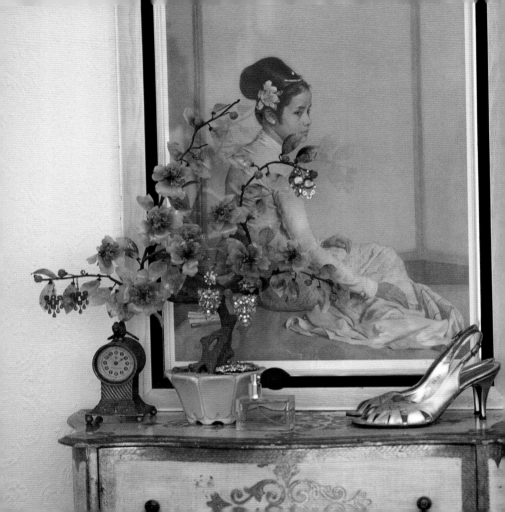

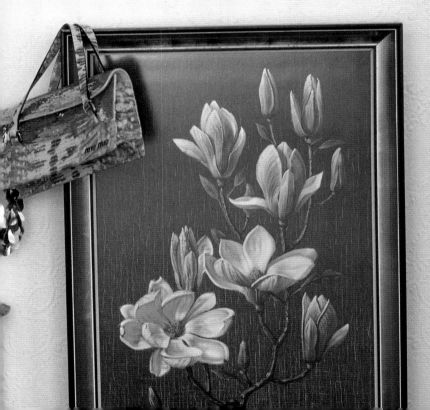

oriental

alluring aromas

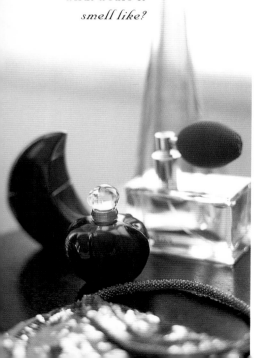

If there were a magic potion for love, what would it smell like?

The oriental family of ingredients – rich in spices, woods, amber and vanilla – are seductive, sultry and overtly sexy.

Romance and seduction in perfumery is, of course, all linked to memory and association. Sensuality is conjured up by many things, but the orientals, with their warm, sweet, heady notes, conjure up heat, power and passionate moments, often creating a cloud of mystery.

The oriental user is a woman who knows how to use her femininity for the utmost impact. Yet sometimes quite shy women like orientals, too. The vanilla note gives her the feeling of sensuality mixed with the memory of a carefree childhood and mother's kitchen.

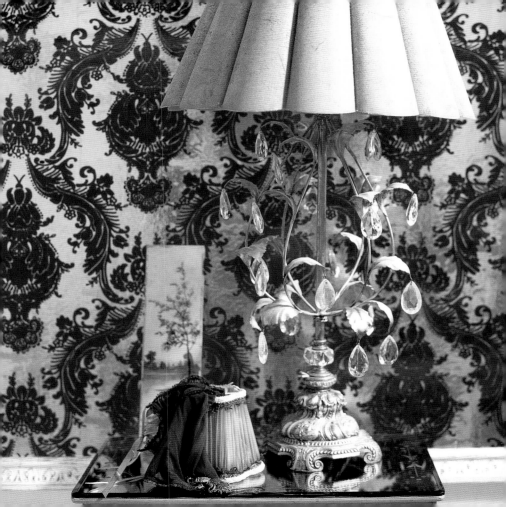

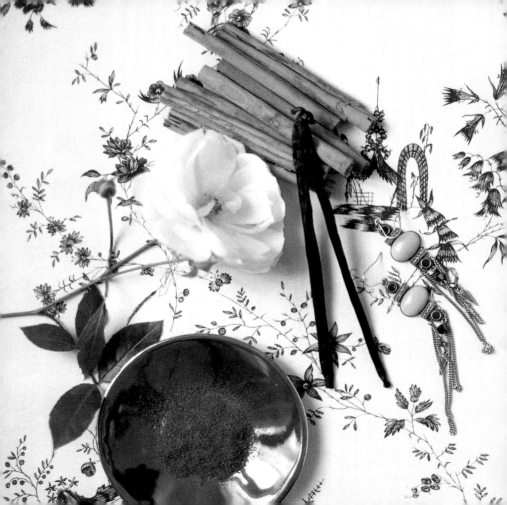

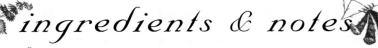

ingredients & notes

Orientals that centre on animalic notes are overtly sexy, strong and enduring. Gourmand (foody) orientals feature vanilla and may contain other distinctive food notes such as chocolate and caramel, while lighter more transparent orientals are blended with heady white flowers and luscious fruits.

VANILLA The key ingredient in any oriental fragrance, vanilla has universal appeal. Its aroma reminds us of the security of childhood. Baby powder is vanilla-scented and some believe that a mother's milk contains chemicals similar to vanilla, which is why we feel content and safe whenever we smell it. And comfort is something we are all looking for when the world around us feels insecure.

Vanilla is a psychogenic aphrodisiac, which means that it works on the central nervous system, exciting all sensation of pleasure.

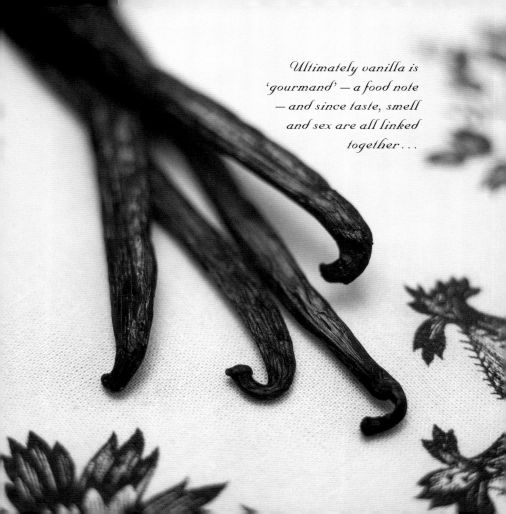

Ultimately vanilla is 'gourmand' — a food note — and since taste, smell and sex are all linked together . . .

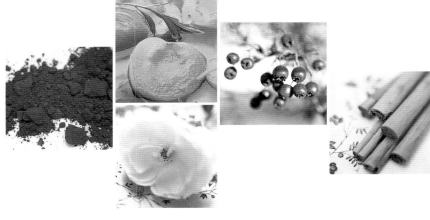

AMBER (or labdanum, its synthetic copy)
An important oily resin used in
perfumery, which smells similar to
ambergris (previously extracted from
whales). The resin gives an animalic,
salty oceanic note to a fragrance. It has
a very sexy, wild impact on scent.
According to legend, Casanova used to
grate ambergris onto his cup of chocolate
each evening before making love.
The association has long been with
chocolate, but perhaps ambergris is
the true aphrodisiac.

ANIMAL NOTES Notes such as civet,
musk, castoreum and ambergris add an
extraordinary richness, warmth and
sensuality to perfume. Animal notes
are akin to the body's own aroma –
especially musk (it contains the same
molecule as humans, called indole).
Naturally it makes sense that applying a
fragrance containing one of these
ingredients intensifies our body's sexual
signals. Blending animal notes with
flower and plant essences simply
enriches the message.

oriental classics

If you like orientals, try:

Ysatis by Givenchy

Very Valentino
by Valentino

Shocking by
Schiaparelli Boucheron

Casmir by Chopard

Poison by Christian Dior

Angel by Dolce
& Gabbana

Coco by Chanel

Youth Dew
by Estée Lauder

Samsara by Guerlain

Must de Cartier

SHALIMAR BY GUERLAIN

Rumour has it that one day Jacques Guerlain absent-mindedly tipped a large quantity of synthetic vanilla into a bottle of Jicky just to see what would happen. The result was Shalimar, the most oriental of perfumes.

When I use vanilla, I get crème caramel. When Jacques [Guerlain] uses vanilla, he gets Shalimar.

ERNEST BEAUX, PERFUMER & CREATOR OF CHANEL NO 5

OPIUM BY YSL

Since its birth in 1977, Opium – a smoky, peppery, spicy oriental scent – has been shrouded in controversy. The American Federal Justice Department tried to have the perfume outlawed, while in other countries it had to be imported under a pseudonym (due to drug import laws), then relabelled once safely in the country. Today the exquisite opiate of a scent is still considered a cult classic.

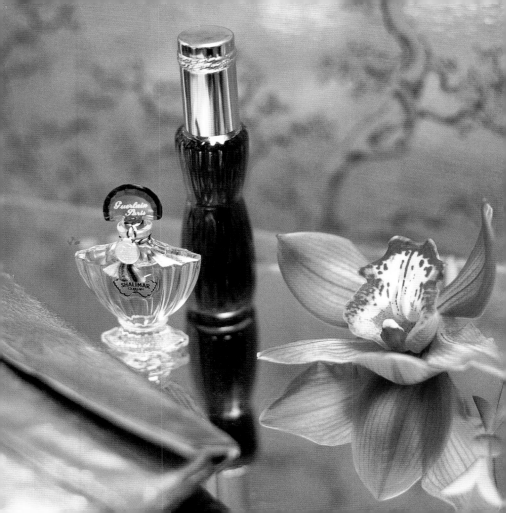

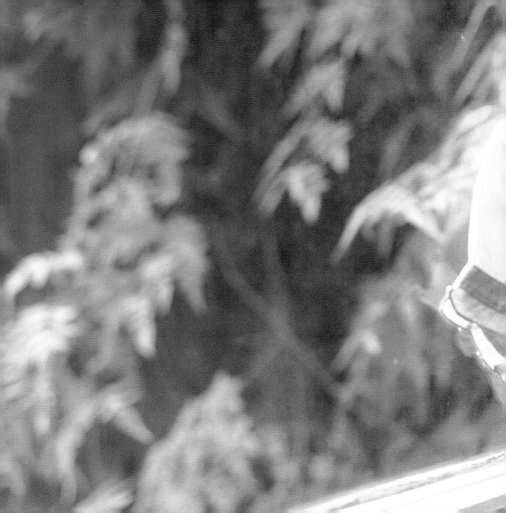

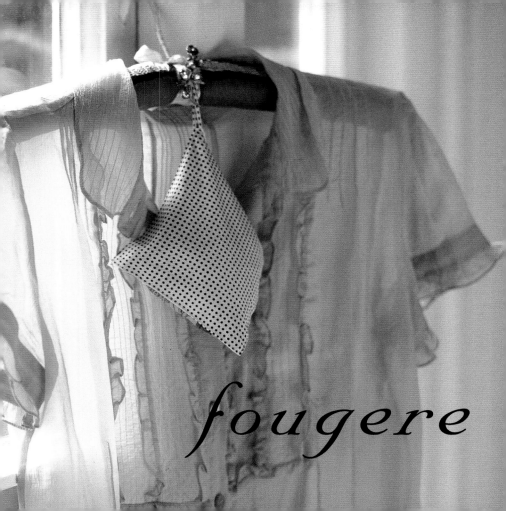

fougere

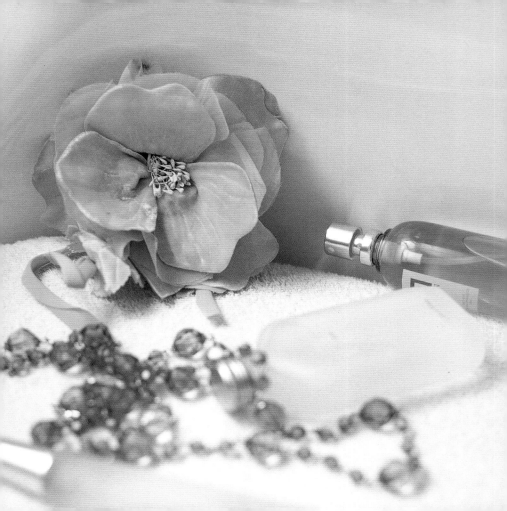

fern-fresh

Ah, beauty in nature. Do crisp winter walks far outweigh the summer sun? When a woman loves the forest, is it the crisp, earthy freshness of the pine needles underfoot, or the sense of danger and mystery?

Fougere, meaning 'fern' in French, was the very first fragrance category to be created. Starting with Jicky by Guerlain in 1889, this category became the home of eau de Cologne, and unisex scents. Now often referred to as herbaceous and green, Hesperidian, fougeres also gave rise to the much-loved chypres and orientals, as this refreshing woodland family share many deep and dusky notes such as oakmoss, patchouli, woods and resins in its base. Indeed, perfumers today, often call the fougere family 'semi-orientals'.

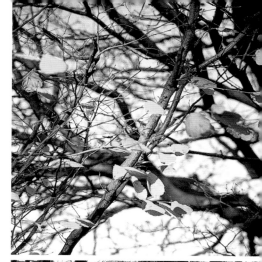

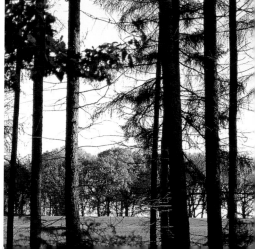

ingredients & notes

Fragrances in this category have a fresh, erotic, woodland
scent, with aromatic herbs (lavender and rosemary),
Hesperidian citrus notes, coumarin and a base of oakmoss,
patchouli and labdanum.

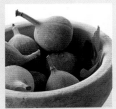

LAVENDER Its distinctive peppery scent is clean and fresh
and reveals the antiseptic qualities of lavender from its tiny
green pods that sit on either side of the purple flowers. It
has been one of the most popular herbs in Britain since the
sixteenth century. Lavender should be gathered in July or
August, just before the flowers have fully opened.

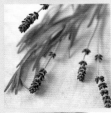

ROSEMARY Who among us wouldn't recognize the distinctive
'camphor-like' fragrance of rosemary? It is rich in fragrant
oil, which is released into the air in the sunshine or warm
breeze whenever you brush against it. Its name is taken from
the Latin *ros marinus*, meaning 'dew of the sea', and it is the
prime ingredient in eau de Cologne.

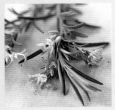

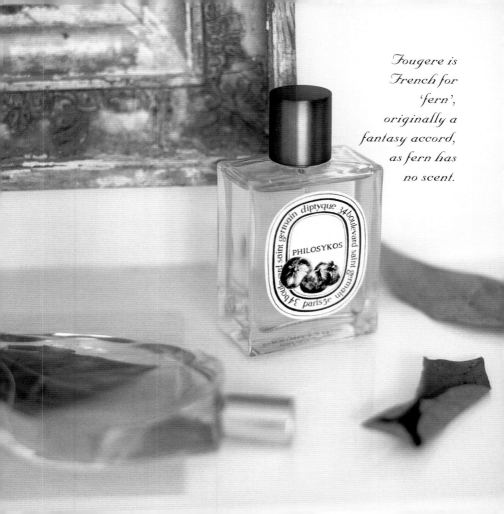

Fougère is French for 'fern', originally a fantasy accord, as fern has no scent.

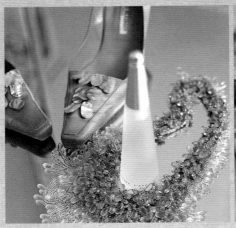
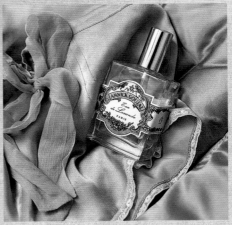

PATCHOULI The epitome of a damp, mossy forest floor, patchouli is a key ingredient for any fougere or chypre fragrance, especially men's. Made popular in the 1960s to mask the aroma of marijuana, it dates back to the early 1800s, when it was used to deter insects from shawls imported from India.

MINT Few modern herbal scents would exist without mint. Discovered in 1700 by botanist John Rea, there are many varieties including peppermint, spearmint and eau de Cologne mint. Its distinctive scent makes it a favourite for adding a fresh note. Research reveals that its uplifting aroma also has a consistent and reliable effect on our ability to concentrate.

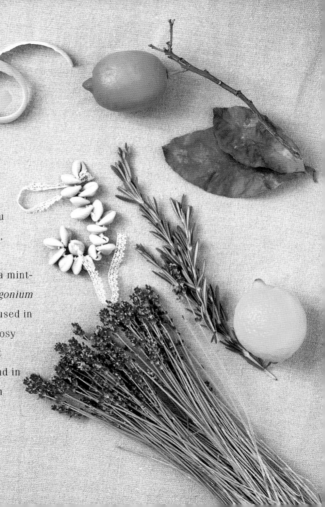

COUMARIN The remarkable smell of freshly mown hay. A synthetic derivative from the tonka bean.

GERANIUM If you crush the geranium leaf under your nail, you instantly capture its sweet, warm, fresh aroma. There are many varieties and they can vary from a mint-like scent to citrus or rose. *Pelargonium capitatum* is the type most often used in cosmetics and perfumery for its rosy scent. This is due to an ingredient called geraniol, which is also found in roses and is frequently used as an alternative to rose.

classic fougere

If you like fougere, try;

4711 by Muelhens

CK One
by Calvin Klein

Bulgari Eau
Parfumee by Bulgari

Acqua di Parma

Wrappings
by Clinique

Eau d'Hadrien
by Annick Goutal

English Lavender
by Yardley

Vetiver by Guerlain

Fougere Royale
by Houbigant

JICKY BY GUERLAIN

Jicky was the first, original fougere fragrance ever created and the forerunner of all 'unisex' fragrances to come. It features familiar eau de Cologne top notes of lavender, bergamot, lemon, mint, thyme, rosemary, a warm heart of coumarin and an amber base with musk and sandalwood. Created for women in 1889, Jicky was simply too racy for the Victorians, who liked women to smell of flowers, so men wore it. It wasn't until the free-spirited 1920s that women sought liberty and independence, and took Jicky back for themselves. Men and women have shared the scent ever since.

EAU SAUVAGE BY CHRISTIAN DIOR

Since its launch in 1966, Eau Sauvage by Christian Dior has been considered 'an aristocrat among perfumes'. The modern classic cologne for men, but equally loved by women, its spicy citrus top notes of lemon, bergamot, basil and cumin mingled with a fresh green derivative of jasmine called hedione that had never been smelt before.

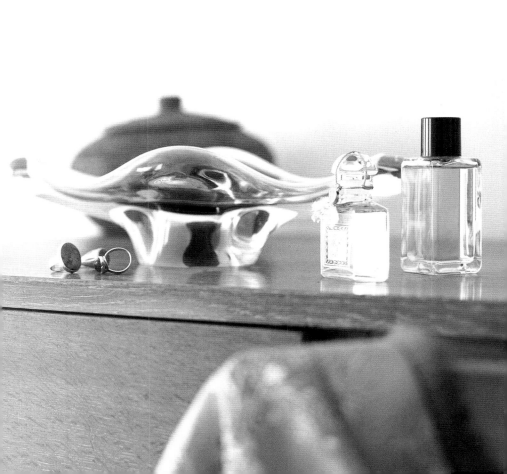

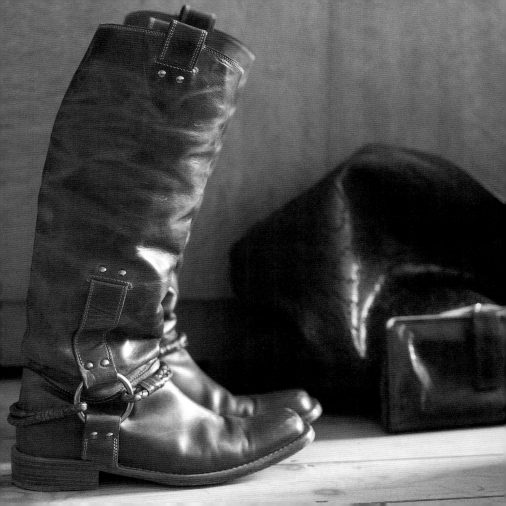

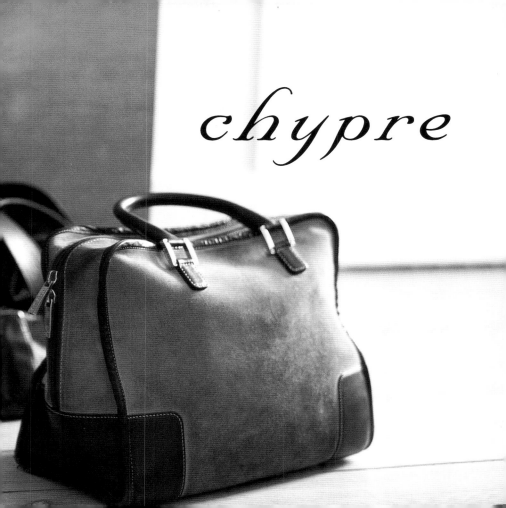

chypre

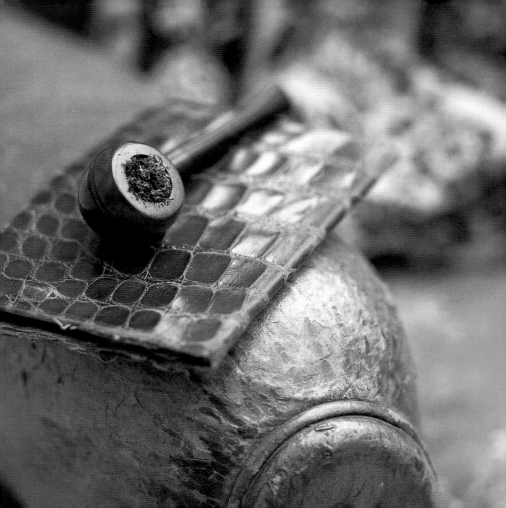

enduring elegance

For me this is the category that defines sophistication and elegance. It is the mother of all scent categories.

The chypre-wearer is a woman whose presence is always felt. She is self-assured, understated and quintessentially elegant. Her attitude to life is black and white – grey and wishy-washy are not in her vocabulary. She is often a person who is very comfortable in her skin. She is grown-up.

Chypre is the kind of intense, deep scent that needs only a dab – never a spray – and that begs to draw one closer to enjoy. It's the left-over base notes that you love in your floral or oriental fragrance – the scent that's left behind once all the obvious juicy, flowery top and middle notes have long gone. Chypres are almost 100 per cent base. Chypre lingers longest, and mingles the most with your own body chemistry. How can you not be affected?

When choosing a lifelong mate, 'Most men don't really like overtly heavy, cloying fruits and flowers,' says Roja Dove. 'Overt is great on "fantasy women", where everything is on show and nothing is left to the imagination; but on a woman they want to share their life with? Always remember: whilst the overt oriental and floral notes promise, the chypres truly deliver.'

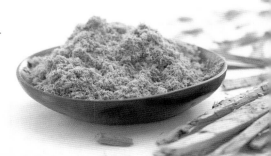

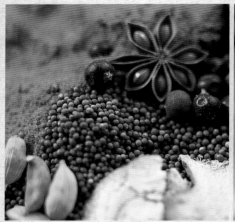
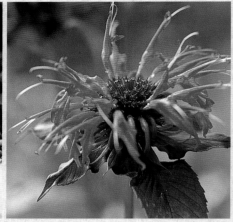

ingredients & notes

This is a highly original group of fragrances based on the contrast between bergamot-type top notes and mossy base notes.

Often strong, spicy and powdery at once, with resins in the base, there are almost as many masculine chypre fragrances as there are feminine ones. The name chypre (pronounced 'shee-pray') originated from the first Coty's Chypre, created in 1917. Its citrus fruits, geranium (often found in this category), spices and oakmoss were so individual that it inspired a whole category of fragrance.

BERGAMOT A divine fresh, lemony herby aroma that may be more recognizable as the smell and flavour of Earl Grey tea. In aromatherapy it is energizing, a tonic, and in perfumery it adds dynamism to the top note, lingering for but a short time, until the fragrance warms round to the heart and soul in the base.

CITRUS Lemon, mandarin, grapefruit – classic eau de Cologne notes shared by men and women alike.

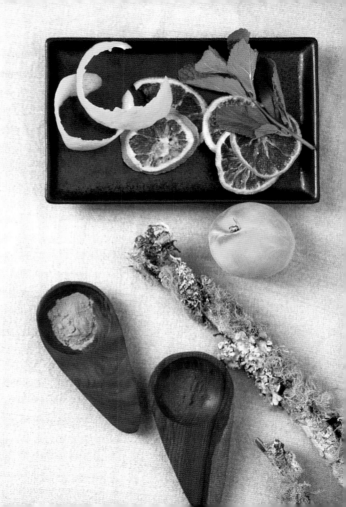

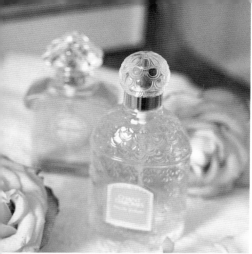

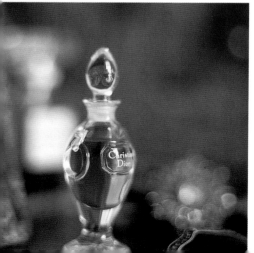

OAKMOSS Extracted from the lichen plant, oakmoss offers an extraordinary creamy, damp, woodland aspect to perfumery, and for that reason can also be found in abundance in fougere fragrances too.

RESINS Myrrh, frankincense, opopanax, galbanum, benzoin and labdanum create a long-lasting base and soul to a perfume, and are very much present in chypre and oriental fragrances. Often referred to as the most ancient ingredients in perfumery, they have been used for centuries in high temples and religious ceremonies.

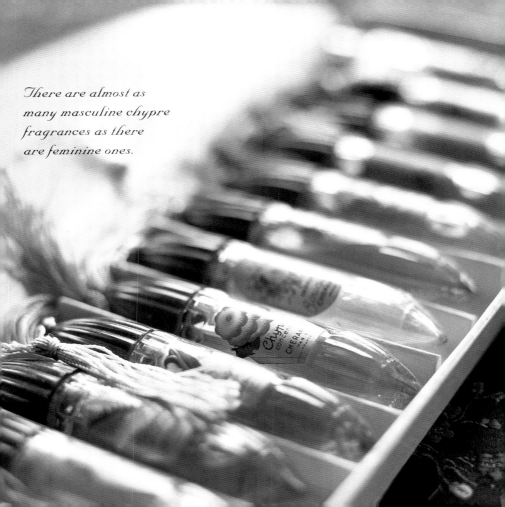

There are almost as
many masculine chypre
fragrances as there
are feminine ones.

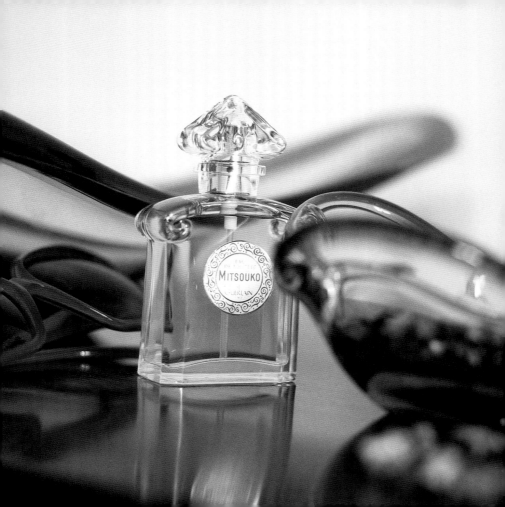

classic chypre

If you like chypre, try:

Ysatis by Givenchy

Miss Dior by Dior

Coriandre
by Jean Couturier

Tabac Blond
by Caron

Aromatics Elixir by
Clinique

La Perla
by La Perla

Paloma Picasso

No 19 by Chanel

MITSOUKO BY GUERLAIN

In Japanese, the name means 'mystery' and the fragrance has been described as 'the way God intended women to smell'. Are you getting the picture? Mitsouko is the scent I need in my life, and I've worn nothing else – save aromatherapy oils – ever since becoming a mother myself so that now when my children snuggle up close, they say I smell of 'home'. This makes the scent all the more poignant for me now, as it will be for them in the future. It's a deeply sensual fragrance. In my heart it's irreplaceable. If you love chypres, you will certainly love Mitsouko.

FEMME BY ROCHAS

A fruity chypre, Femme is voluptuous and womanly in every way. Tantalizing notes of cinnamon-coated sugarplums, juicy peaches and crystallized prunes, a heavy floral heart of jasmine and rose, and a sultry base of amber, oakmoss and musk... It's pure sex in a bottle. Even the curvaceous shape of Femme's original bottle was inspired by Mae West's hips, and the box once came dressed in black Chantilly lace.

useful addresses

STOCKISTS & STORES

ANNICK GOUTAL
www.annickgoutal.nl

BOOTS
www.wellbeing.com
Over 4,000 stores nationwide.

CHANEL
www.chanel.com

CHRISTIAN DIOR
www.dior.com

DIPTYQUE
195 Westbourne Grove
London W11 2SB
t. 020 7727 8673
www.diptyque.tm.fr

ESTEE LAUDER
www.esteelauder.com

GARDEN PHARMACY
119 Long Acre
Covent Garden
London WC2E 9PB
t. 020 7836 1007

GUERLAIN
www.guerlain.com

HOUSE OF FRASER
www.houseoffraser.co.uk

ISSEY MIYAKE
www.isseymiyake.com

JO MALONE
www.jomalone.com

KENZO
www.kenzo.com

NINA RICCI
www.ninaricci.com

PRADA
www.prada.com

VERA WANG
www.verawang.com

BUSINESS CREDITS

EMMA CASSI
www.emmacassi.com
t.020 8487 2836

**FLORENCE TORRENS
& PAUL FRITH**
For details/bookings contact
paul@paulfrith.co.uk

**JOSEPHINE RYAN
ANTIQUES**
63 Abbeville Road
London SW4 9JW
t/f. 020 8675 3900
www.josephineryanantiques.co.uk

MAISONETTE
79 Chamberlayne Road
London NW10 3ND
Opening hours (Tues–Sat)
11.00–18.00
Contact Amanda Sellers
& Martin Barrell
t. 020 8964 8444
f. 020 8964 8464
www.maisonette.uk.com
maisonetteUK@aol.com

MARIANNE COTTERILL
The Lounge at Selfridges
t. 020 8931 6649
www.loungeonline.net

SPINA
12 Kingsgate Place
London NW6 4TA
t. 020 7328 5274
f. 020 7624 2078
www.spinadesign.co.uk
spinadesign@btconnect.com

picture credits

All photography by Claire Richardson
Key: ph= photographer, a=above, b=below,
r=right, l=left, c=centre.

Page 1 Josephine Ryan's house in London; 2 & 7 Marianne Cotterill's house in London – products available from The Lounge at Selfridges; 8 Florence & Paul's Edwardian house in London; 11 Josephine Ryan's house in London; 17 Emma Cassi's flat in London; designs by Emma Cassi; 20–22 Florence & Paul's Edwardian house in London; 23 Spina (tie-backs, tassels & crystal installations) private showroom – by appointment only; 24a Amanda Sellers and Martin Barrell's flat in North West London; 26l, alc & cr ph David Montgomery; 27 Josephine Ryan's house in London; 28–29 Marianne Cotterill's house in London – products available from The Lounge at Selfridges; 30 Josephine Ryan's house in London; 32–33 Amanda Sellers and Martin Barrell's flat in North West London; 34 Florence & Paul's Edwardian house in London; 35 Marianne Cotterill's house in London – products available from The Lounge at Selfridges; 36–37 Emma Cassi's flat in London; designs by Emma Cassi; 39l ph Debi Treloar; 39alc ph William Lingwood; 41 Marianne Cotterill's house in London – products available from The Lounge at Selfridges; 42–44 Amanda Sellers and Martin Barrell's flat in North West London; 46 ph Peter Cassidy; 47 Emma Cassi's flat in London; designs by Emma Cassi; 48 Marianne Cotterill's house in London – products available from The Lounge at Selfridges; 50–53 Florence & Paul's Edwardian house in London; 54 Marianne Cotterill's house in London – products available from The Lounge at Selfridges; 55 ph David Montgomery; 56l ph James Merrell; 56r ph Caroline Arber; 58a Spina (tie-backs, tassels & crystal installations) private showroom – by appointment only; 58b & 60 Amanda Sellers and Martin Barrell's flat in North West London.

acknowledgments

This book is dedicated to my late mother and father. On a daily basis
I am happy to be reminded of them by the many scents and pleasures
around me. Always missed, but never forgotten.

This little book is a culmination of stories and quotes handed over to me
during my many years in beauty journalism. Perfume is often intangible,
only captured through emotional moments and experiences, and learning
that in itself was only made possible by the following wonderful people:
my dear Roja Dove, never a perfume piece could be penned without
words from this master of perfumery; aromatherapist and perfumer
Glenda Taylor of Enata, Jo Malone, Lyn Harris, Richard Harris of
Guerlain. Love and thanks to my darling friend Kate Hudson. I'd also
like to thank all the many fragrance PRs who kindly gave me information
and lent precious bottles for photography.

For bespoke fragrance consultation, contact Roja Dove, Perfumer and
Creator of Roja Dove Haute Parfumerie, Urban Retreat, 5th Floor,
Harrods; and Glenda Taylor at www.enata.co.uk.

Further fragrant reading:
Perfume Legends by Michael Edwards, H M Éditions, 1996
Perfume by Patrick Suskind, Vintage, 2001
The Emperor of Scent by Chandler Burr, Random House, 2003